MALTODEXTRIN: A SILENT FOOD KILLER

By

Dr. Ashish Srivastava

TABLE OF CONTENTS

Chapter 1 : Introduction

In a fast-paced world like today, what to eat often takes its cue from convenience. More and more of our diet is now being this way and isn't merely pre-packaged snacks - it's food ready to put in the microwave, heat up or eat straight from the supermarket shelf. Where there is convenience however there's also hidden costs: our health.

There is an ingredient that goes unnoticed by most of us, though found in almost every kind of sports drink and gluten-free product. It is Maltodextrin -- despite advertising to the contrary safe for human consumption on their/its packaging without further qualification beyond all the hype, the hard truth is this: although Maltodextrin has been given clean bills of health and is "natural," that doesn't mean there aren't some very real complications to deal with it.

But what makes Maltodextrin so fearful? Firstly, it's highly processed. By a series of processing stages involving extensive chemical modification and the removal of all nutrients, from starches like corn, rice or potato some Maltodextrin is obtained.

What's left after this process is a refined sugar -like substance with a high glycemic index (GI), meaning that when entering your body through food or drink it will cause blood sugar to jump almost immediately? This can be especially bad for people who have diabetes and insulin resistance (problems using their own naturally occurring insulin). General blood sugar spikes over time can make you gain weight, cause inflammation in addition to other health issues.

The second hidden danger of Maltodextrin is that it may have an impact on your gut microbiome. There is some emerging research suggesting that it may disturb the delicate equilibrium between good and harmful bacteria residing in our digestive tract. If something goes wrong with the friendly flora down there—via a population swing toward pathogenic species of microbes or something else dire to their natural environment—an unhealthy relationship quickly develops. Yet unlike dietary fibers which people need to maintain life-sustaining functions, Maltodextrin is precisely the opposite: it is a filler body that can make nothing from. But doesn't stop there--Maltodextrin is also widely used in processed foods, including gluten-free and sugar-free options that may be less healthy but those aiming to eat healthily will find it particularly tough going indeed on the one hand, maltodextrin is typically unsigned.

You think that you're making sensible food choices. But if the truth be told, in the long run, eating such a substance can do nothing good for your health. After you've completed this book, you will understand the roots of maltodextrin, its various applications, and the scientific evidence behind why it's just not good for your health. Most importantly, we shall present ways that you can use to find maltodextrin within your diet and instead opt for more healthy alternatives. By the end of it, you'll have knowledge to guard your health and can make sound decisions for your body in the long run.

Chapter 2 : What Is Maltodextrin? A Secret Component

Maltodextrin (a polysaccharide and a type of carbohydrate) is often used as an additive in food. It plays a huge role in food production serving as a thickener, filler, or preservative. However, have you ever thought about what exactly it is and why it's so common in our food amidst all the nutrition transition?

In this chapter we will explain exactly what maltodextrin is and elucidate how it differs from other common carbohydrates. Maltodextrin comes from starches such as corn, rice or potatoes and is processed into a fine white powder. Then they grind this into a fine powder for adding to foods, to aid in texturizing, wanting adherence or shelf life. Being versatile and cheap to produce, is one of the reasons that food manufacturers love it so much. Trends like this teach us to never fear something healthy and easy seems bad, because now you even make a product but that's not good for health.

The main issue with maltodextrin is that it's incredibly processed. In the making process, enzymes and acids assist in breaking down the starch into smaller segments. That process removes all of the nutritional value, and all that is left at the end -- a highly perishable substance that has no fiber or vitamins.

So whenever you eat foods that contain maltodextrin, in essence what you are doing is consuming nothing but empty calories -- which have the potential to send your blood glucose soaring suddenly. This kind of abrupt increase can be extremely dangerous for people with diabetes, yet it also creates long-term problems for those who are healthy.

And not only does maltodextrin have a high glycemic index; it also damages the health of your gut. The human gut is home to trillions of bacteria living in a delicate balance that are vital for digestion, immunity, and overall health. Some studies suggest that maltodextrin can change the balance of these bacteria, tilting the scale toward harmful pathogens while reducing the number of beneficial bacteria living there. This imbalance is liable to cause digestive problems, inflammation, and perhaps even such chronic diseases as inflammatory bowel disease (IBD). Nevertheless, maltodextrin is ubiquitous and it can even appear in foods that are considered healthy. In other words, you might still be consuming maltodextrin even if you are trying to eat cleanly. It is used as a source of orally administered fluids unless significant portions of maltodextrin are consumed along with vitamin-free water's caloric value would be so much that energy would provide makes fasting unnecessary or medically ill-advised for example many oral rehydration solutions for children is only 40% glucose being replaced' using the standard empirical experimental preparation.- it also gives gluten-free food products often known to use maltodextrin as its substitute --while sugar-free and low-fat products may contain maltodextrins flavor enhancing properties.

The next chapter will also tell you about the production process of maltodextrin and how we should read it in the ingredient list. You need to find out where your food has maltodextrin, and here is how you can reduce its intake while securing your health.

Chapter 3 : Production Process of Maltodextrin

Maltodextrin may be a simple looking ingredient, but the steps to make maltodextrin are not so straightforward. If you want to know why maltodextrin can be so bad for your health, it all starts with understanding how they make the stuff. Though it is extracted from plant based sources such as corn, rice, and potatoes The process converts a whole food into an isolated powder through many chemical processes that essentially render the product nutritionally void. Touching upon the natural origins of maltodextrin, and ending with the super processed, chemical found within all your favorite foods. And the journey of this nasty compound like maltodextrin will give you an idea of just how much harm it has started to cause in your body.

The Starch Source

Maltodextrin is typically produced from a grain, which may be in the form of corn, wheat, rice, or potatoes. The choice is sometimes based on regional availability and manufacturer preference. In the United States, it is more likely to be derived based on corn because the crop is readily available and less expensive to produce. Consumers may, however, be adversely affected because most of the corn grown in U.S. fields are genetically modified (GMO), which can have negative implications on the quality and safety of the starch made.

Hydrolysis: Breaking Down the Starch

Hydrolysis is the subsequent step in producing maltodextrin. In this step, the complex starch is broken down into smaller carbohydrate molecules by enzymes or acids. This is necessary because raw starch molecules are too big and thus too complicated to cater for all the demands that food producers demand. Hydrolysis breaks down starch molecules into shorter chains of glucose, yielding a substance that can easily be water-dissolved, thickened, or sweetened.

Hydrolysis strips the starch of any fiber or nutrients it once contained, leaving it something only good for functional purposes—texture, preservation, and sometimes taste. This process of refining is the reason maltodextrin contains no nutritional value, hence its moniker "empty calories."

Spray Drying and Milling

After the starch has been broken down to a more basic carbohydrate unit through hydrolysis, the solution undergoes another process which is spray-drying. The hydrolyzed starch solution is sprayed upon a fine, white powder known as maltodextrin. Such a powder can be mixed into many processed foods without altering their taste profiles, hence food manufacturers enjoy it so much. The process of spray-drying then removes the remaining moisture from the end product, hence shelf stability over extended periods.

This is the main reason maltodextrin is used widely in packaged and processed foods: its long shelf life is an important asset for mass production.

The Chemical Change

At this point, maltodextrin is considerably changed. While it originally derives from natural starch, enzymes or acids used in hydrolysis, along with the extreme heat that is applied during spray-drying, ensure it is indistinguishable from its origin. Such big starch molecules have been broken down into very much smaller chains, largely glucose units, which now function as if they were sugar rather than a complex carbohydrate.

The high glycemic index resulting from the chemical behavior of maltodextrin makes foods quite unhealthy. Foods that have a high GI are absorbed by the body rapidly and, as such, quickly raise the blood sugar levels. It is very essential to the diabetic and non-diabetic individuals in terms of constant peaks in their blood sugar since constant peaks might cause long-term health issues that could cause one to suffer with obesity, inflammation, or metabolic disorders.

Additives and GMO Concerns

Many types of maltodextrin are manufactured from genetically modified (GMO) crops, and the crop most likely used in the United States is corn. Most of the corn consumed in food systems is genetically engineered to be pest- and herbicide-resistant and may well potentially also cause health impacts through its ingestion of these modified substances. It lies in the source crop's quality and the chemical process it goes through to create maltodextrin.

Moreover, in its manufacture, some maltodextrin could be mixed up with other additives or preservatives or stabilizers to make the malt work for inclusion in other food items. These are not often listed separately on food ingredient lists, leaving consumers oblivious to the totality of chemicals they are ingesting.

Industrial Applications of Maltodextrin

This compound, maltodextrin, is also industrial friendly. It is applied both in the food industry and in the cosmetic and pharmaceutical fields besides its industrial applications. In the pharmaceutical field, this compound has a wide usage as a filler or binder for medicine preparations and supplements. Due to neutral taste and good solubility, it can easily mix to formulate pills and powders. This chemical serves as a thickener or an emulsifier within cosmetics, like lotions and creams, to mix oil and water-based ingredients well.

While harmless in non-food products, that is as widespread as it is troubling this much it has become a part of everyday life. This led many to question just how much of this heavily processed substance many have been dosed with regularly without even realizing it.

Disconnection Between Natural and Processed

Ultimately, the disconnection between maltodextrin's natural roots and processed result is the biggest problem. It starts off as a carbohydrate, but by the extensive refining process, it becomes something very far from what nature had intended. This transformation points out why maltodextrin is problematic. Though it may technically start off as something natural, its highly processed state generally creates problems in the human body, especially if it's taken in copious amounts.

Most of the consumers have been duped to believe that maltodextrin is a carbohydrate. Though chemically, it is one, in human physiology, it behaves more like sugar. That is because maltodextrin has a high glycemic index and gets absorbed into the system within no time. Compared to complicated carbohydrates, maltodextrin is not something that fuels slowly for a long period. Maltodextrin does not have any nutritional benefits compared to complex carbohydrates. It does not contain fiber, vitamins, or minerals as its sources are usually extracted from wheat and other whole grains, fruits, and vegetables.

Why Do You Need to Know About the Process?

Knowing how maltodextrin is made makes you realize rather quickly why it can be so dangerous. All the chemical processing really removes any beneficial qualities, and all you're left with is something that's not only nutritionally empty but potentially toxic in big quantities. Understanding how often maltodextrin hides in so many foods-sauces, dressings, gluten-free or sports drinks, you quickly see why being mindful of what's in your food is a big deal.

In maltodextrin, the power of this development lies in the demonstration of how large parts of modern diets are dominated by highly processed foods. What once used to be natural and wholesome ingredients can be transformed into dangers through industrial manufacturing processes. Convenience for food manufacturers often presents a disadvantage to the consumer's long-term health.

In the following chapter, we'll take a closer look at exactly how ubiquitously maltodextrin appears in the modern food supply-and exactly what kinds of products it's most likely to turn up in-and why making healthy choices is still such a challenge.

Chapter 4 : Maltodextrin Is In Everything You Eat

Till now, you are well-informed about the maltodextrin and how it is produced and obtained. So where do people find this stuff ? Any ideas ? Maltodextrin is one of the most widely used additive agents for processed foods, found in products you'd never expect.

In this chapter you learn how maltodextrin is used ubiquitously in processed foods and drinks. The range includes such ubiquitous items as snack foods and frozen meals; protein powders; and even so-called "health" products. You'll learn to recognize it on ingredient labels and learn why food manufacturers are so enamored of its use.

Maltodextrin in Packaged and Processed Foods

Most grocery center products contain some kind of processed additive, and maltodextrin is one of the most common. It's frequently a thickening agent in sauces, soups, or salad dressings but is also found in instant food like mashed potatoes and rice preparations. Since maltodextrin dissolves well and has a neutral taste, it can usually be added to almost any type of food product without affecting the flavor.

A filler or preservative in snack foods, maltodextrin extends the shelf life of chips and crackers and many other packaged goods. In fact, even frozen meals-something many are resorting to for convenience-incorporate maltodextrin to optimize texture and ensure flavor after freezing and subsequent heating.

Hidden in "Healthy" Foods

What is alarming about maltodextrin's widespread availability is its frequent appearance on allegedly healthy foods. Gluten-free, low-fat, or sugar-free foods frequently rely on maltodextrin to replace other ingredients. For instance, gluten-free products may necessitate maltodextrin as a binder or thickener: how the busy consumer typically purchasing processed foods can hardly ever notice this?.

Maltodextrin is also a common constituent of sports drinks and protein powders. These products are often marketed to athletes, weightlifters, and fitness-conscious consumers as something "healthy," but they deliver high levels of fast-digesting sugars in the form of maltodextrin.

We will certainly dig into specific food and food groups that often contain maltodextrin, why it's used so extensively, and offer practical information on how to decipher food labels to do it better in your diet.

Chapter 5 : Maltodextrin and Blood Sugar: A Severe Spike

One of the health concerns with maltodextrin is its impact on blood sugar levels. Although it is one of the most popular food additives, its effect on human bodies could be much worse than you ever imagined. Since maltodextrin is so refined, it appears quickly in the blood and causes a high rise in levels of blood glucose. It is a serious issue in the people diagnosed with diabetes or who may easily acquire insulin resistance. More or repeated blood sugar spiking can culminate in more chronic health issues, such as obesity and even heart diseases, among healthy individuals.

We're going to dive deeper into how maltodextrin affects your blood sugar, compare it to other carbohydrates, and explore why the high glycemic index of maltodextrin makes it particularly toxic. We will also delve into the cumulative effects of multiple blood sugar peaks on your body and provide you with some practical actions to help minimize the risk.

You recall learning about the glycemic index of sugar- that scoring, from 0-100, of how foods affect your blood sugar. But, like sugar, maltodextrin is a short-chain carbohydrate, meaning it breaks down during digestion very quickly into glucose which spikes your blood sugar.

In order to get a good understanding of how maltodextrin would work on blood sugar, one needs to understand what glycemic index is. GI is a measure used to rank carbohydrates from 'how quickly they raise blood sugar levels'. Foods whose constituent GI values are high are broken down and absorbed quickly, therefore resulting in an immediate increase in blood sugar, whereas foods with a low GI are absorbed more slowly with a gradual increase in glucose.

Maltodextrin has an excessively high GI—it's much higher than even common ordinary table sugar, with some estimates indicating its GI at between 85 and 105. For proper perspective, a food is said to have a high GI if it scores over 70, and it's common to suggest avoiding or taking it in moderation, especially for those that are controlling their blood sugar levels.

How Maltodextrin Causes High Spikes in Blood Sugar Level

The digestion process makes maltodextrin breakdown fats into glucose, which easily becomes the simplest form of sugar. It is so refined that your body does not have to work so much to break it down. Such rapid digestion will send glucose racing into your bloodstream and cause your blood sugar level to spike up suddenly.

The release causes your pancreas to have a hormone called insulin. This hormone enables glucose movement from your blood into your cells, which either exhaust the glucose for energy or store it as fat. In a healthy individual, this system will work fine. Still, the rapid rise in glucose can squeeze your pancreas to release more insulin than usual, resulting in a catastrophic drop in blood sugar later on. That rises and falls in blood sugar levels cause you to feel tired, cranky, and wanting more sugar or carbs-it essentially lays the groundwork for a vicious cycle of overeating and poor energy control.

Maltodextrin and Diabetes

In people with diabetes and even those prediabetic, the risks of maltodextrin may be even more pronounced. Diabetes is simply the inability of an individual to regulate his blood glucose levels and this may be due either to a complete lack of insulin, known as type 1 diabetes, or a body that resists insulin, called type 2 diabetes. Foods with high GI values like maltodextrin increase one's blood sugar level precariously and hence make it difficult for a diabetic person to control his or her blood sugar level. These spines may lead to hyperglycemia-high blood sugar-and, potentially, over many years, to complications involving diabetes: nerve damage, kidney disease, and cardiovascular disease.

Maltodextrin has been found to create insulin resistance in people who are not detected with diabetes. Insulin resistance means that the body is resistant to insulin. With time, this can lead to diabetes type 2 because the pancreas cannot absorb the overproduction of more insulin to try to control blood sugar.

Maltodextrin's Role in Weight Gain and Obesity

Blood sugar spikes caused by maltodextrin do not only pose a health risk to diabetics but tend to cause weight gain and obesity in normal individuals. In such scenarios where your body responds to high blood sugar by releasing large amounts of insulin, all the glucose that is not immediately used for energy is stored as fat. These foods will, in the long run, add up to more body fats, mainly on the abdomen; this is risky for a high risk of diseases that are brought about by metabolism.

Another change is the very rapid blood sugar fluctuations, whereby your system may feel hungry within an hour or so after you have eaten, which actually might be because the sharp decrease in blood sugar after the high spike created gives your brain a signal that it needs more food even though calories have already been taken in. This creates hunger and cravings for more high-carb or sugary foods, thus perpetuating a cycle of poor dietary choices and weight gain.

How Maltodextrin Compares to Other Carbohydrates

All carbs are not equal in blood sugar spiking. Complex carb sources such as whole grains, fruits, and vegetables have a more gradual effect because they contain fiber, which slows glucose from getting into the bloodstream rapidly. The low-GI foods take a longer time to get digested slowly thereby providing a sustained release of energy and blood sugars stay in the stable zone throughout the day.

On the contrary, maltodextrin has an immediate effect like simple sugars, which are digested and get absorbed very quickly. Being a carbohydrate, it might be mentioned on the ingredient list; however, the impact it creates for your body is very close to the same as consuming refined sugar, which can make it even more destructive for those who would keep their blood sugar within the normal level or planning to lose some weight.

Cumulative Effects of Blood Sugar Spikes

While acute effects-the immediate onset of fatigue, hunger, and irritability-are rather obvious, repercussions of repeated fluctuations of blood sugar over a larger canvas are much more subtle yet far more dangerous. Repeated elevation of blood sugar levels causes chronic inflammation in the body, contributing to many other diseases, such as cardiovascular disease, cancer, and neurodegenerative diseases like Alzheimer's.

High blood sugar spikes may, over time, lead to a medical condition referred to as insulin resistance. This happens because your cells will start responding inadequately to the hormone; hence, you will struggle increasingly to control the sugar in your body. In the long run, it may cause an overwork of the pancreas and organs, thereby leading you to become a victim of type 2 diabetes. More so, as much as the condition may not be worse than acquiring diabetes, it will always stress the metabolic system, and it may further cause obesity, high cholesterol, and hypertension.

Mitigating the Influence of Maltodextrin on Blood Sugar

Even though it's tough to totally remove maltodextrin from your diet, you can always do some things to try and avoid its impact on blood sugar. A few strategies include the following.

Be Careful Reading Labels: Maltodextrin is usually marked on the ingredients of most packaged and processed food, but it might be quite common for people to miss them. Look out when you read the ingredients of foods that say low-fat, gluten-free, or sugar-free.

Whole Foods: Use as many whole, unprocessed foods as possible. Fruits, vegetables, whole grains, legumes, and lean proteins provide complex carbohydrates, fiber, and essential nutrients, which support blood sugar regulation.

Pair with Protein or Fiber: Pair carbohydrates with protein or fiber when you eat them. Gradual glucose digestion will help maintain more steady levels of blood sugar.

Cut Processed Snacks : Snack foods-many of them are those with chips, crackers, or protein bars containing maltodextrin. Replace them with healthy snacks such as nuts, seeds, or fresh fruits and vegetables.

See a Healthcare Provider: Discuss the options with your doctor or a registered dietitian if you are diagnosed with diabetes or want to get concerns about your blood sugar levels. He/She will assist in creating a meal plan that minimizes high-GI foods like maltodextrin.

Conclusion

Maltodextrin is an additive to food that may be harmless-looking but research has revealed that its impact on blood sugars is profoundly dangerous. Its glycemic index is very high, and its absorption time to the bloodstream is very fast, meaning it can cause high spikes in blood sugar with the danger of weight gain, potential insulin resistance, and sometimes diabetes. By learning the ways in which maltodextrin will affect your body and by reducing your consumption, you will be able to stay healthy and avoid the long-term effects of constant blood sugar fluctuations.

Hidden Danger: How Maltodextrin Affects Your Gut and Digestive Health-More than Meets the Eye

In the next chapter, we continue into more details on how maltodextrin affects your gut and your digestive health-the other dangers posed by this common food additive that is more than just meets the eye.

Chapter 6 : Maltodextrin and Your Gut Health-The Gut Connection

Of course, spiking blood sugar levels are one of the more immediate and noticeable effects of maltodextrin consumption, but its impact on your digestive health can be just as troublesome-though often much more sneaky. Your digestive system, and indeed your gut microbiome in particular, are crucial to your overall health. This rare balance of bacterial and fungal life, and so forth, touches every minute part of our biology-from digestion and immune function to mental health and inflammation. And when it is disrupted-that is, by maltodextrin-the results are far-reaching and severe.

We're going to delve a little deeper into how maltodextrin affects your gut health, how it might contribute to the presence of pathological microbes, and its link to inflammation and a compromised digestive system. It can help you understand how this ubiquitous food additive interacts with the gut and why it's not only a risk for your waistline and blood sugar control but also to your long-term health.

The Gut Microbiome: Your Body's Inner Ecosystem

Before we delve into maltodextrin's direct effects on gut health, let us recall how important the gut microbiome is. Human intestinal tracts harbour an amount estimated to be trillions of microbes-thought of as a collective. These microbes-estimated, include a massive range of bacteria, and with such aid help further break down food and produce vitamins while also serving as a body's defense mechanism against deleterious pathogens. They also regulate the body's immune system and keep inflammation under control.

A healthy gut microbiome is diverse and balanced, yet the helpful bacteria maintain harmful microbes. Poor diet, stress, antibiotics, and some additives such as maltodextrin disrupt that balance and let bad bacteria run wild. Such imbalances have triggered a host of diseases, from inflammation, to digestive disorders, even autoimmunity.

Impact of Maltodextrin on Gut Bacteria

Malotodextrin does have an effect on the bacteria balance in your gut. Among the most alarming results is the fact that maltodextrin fosters the proliferation of harmful bacteria like E. coli and Salmonella. These pathogenic bacteria attach to your gut lining, causing inflammation and increasing the chance of infections.

In one research study, it was revealed that maltodextrin promoted the proliferation of E. coli. In such cases, harmful bacterium E. coli causes severe infections in the intestines. Such a study underlines how the substance maltodextrin makes the biofilm formation easy for harmful bacteria, enabling these to thrive and multiply in the gut with even the body's natural protections. This is very frightening as it implies that consuming maltodextrin can make you more susceptible to gut infections besides chronic digestive issues.

In addition, it has been suggested that maltodextrin inhibits the beneficial gut microflora, like Lactobacillus reuteri, a particular genus of microbes that has been found to be anti-inflammatory. Maltodextrin causes dysbiosis-a microbiome imbalance-that has been linked with these pathologies, such as IBS and IBD, and even autoimmunity.

Inflammation and Gut Disorders

Inflammation is one of the most crucial modes through which maltodextrin acts to regulate gut health. Chronic inflammation remains at the base of most disorders of the digestive system, including Crohn's disease and ulcerative colitis, two conditions considered inflammatory bowel disease, or IBD. In patients with IBD, the immune response begins to attack the lining of the gut, creating a vicious cycle of pain, diarrhea, and all those other absolutely debilitating symptoms.

Research has shown that maltodextrin increases the inflammatory response in pathologies related to the gut, notably in predisposed IBD patients. For instance, maltodextrin causes the proliferation of harmful bacteria while debilitating the beneficial bacteria; such a situation worsens the symptoms of the conditions and makes them harder to manage.

For people with no established digestive issues, long-term consumption of maltodextrin can also cause subtle inflammatory diseases in the gut. Chronic, low-level inflammation is also supposedly harmless-at least in the short term; but it will damage the lining of the gut eventually and likely contribute to subsequent infections, food sensitivities, or even autoimmune diseases.

Role of Maltodextrin in "Leaky Gut" Syndrome

Another alarming effect of maltodextrin on the gut is that it may lead to or at least exacerbate "leaky gut" syndrome, also referred to as increased intestinal permeability. In healthy digestion, the lining of the gut forms a barrier through which some nutrients are allowed into the bloodstream but prevents most of the harmful particles from passing through. When gut integrity is compromised, undigested food particles, toxins, and pathogens breach the gut lining and enter the bloodstream.

This condition has been linked to a wide spectrum of health conditions ranging from autoimmune diseases, chronic fatigue syndrome to even psychiatric disorders. Maltodextrin, therefore enhances the presence of leaky gut through the effects of inflammation and abrasion on the intestines, allowing toxins to freely enter the bloodstream. This is very ominous because it is difficult to diagnose and people face symptoms that are mostly mistaken for other causes such as bloating, fatigue, and food sensitivities.

Association to Autoimmune Disorders

With increasing research, it has been documented that maltodextrin does indeed interact with the gut microbiota to develop autoimmune disorders. Autoimmune disorders refer to those diseases in which the immune system of the individual tends to start a war against the healthy cells found in the body. Many autoimmune disorders have been found to be associated with inflammation as well as alteration of the gut flora. Such diseases include rheumatoid arthritis, lupus, as well as multiple sclerosis. All these diseases have been connected with dysbiosis and leaky gut.

It also causes or exacerbates inflammation and gut bacteria imbalances, and so it can start or worsen autoimmune responses. The susceptibility of the immune system makes such individuals prone to the action of maltodextrin, especially with a genetic predisposition towards autoimmune diseases.

Processed Foods: Maltodextrin is likely to hide within many foods.

Ironically, probably the most intimidating part of maltodextrin is the sheer number of times you'll encounter it on a packaged food. Due to its properties as a thickener, filler, and preservative, a lot of foods that you would think might not contain maltodextrin, such as sauces or dressings or baked goods, and even some "healthy" foods like protein powder and supplements.

To those individuals who still do not see the dangers of maltodextrin, it may easily be consumed in large quantities without the person realizing the effects maltodextrin is having on gut health. Eventually, these chronic digestive problems can result in conditions involving persistent inflammation and a weakened immune system, which hinders one's ability to maintain overall health and wellness.

Protecting Your Gut from Maltodextrin

Though impossible to steer clear of 100%, try these tips to safeguard your gut health and reduce exposure:

Read labels: Inspect ingredient listings for maltodextrin, especially in processed and packaged foods. Be extra vigilant with low-fat, sugar-free, or gluten-free products-many contain maltodextrin as filler.

Choose Whole Foods: The best way to keep your gut in tip-top shape is through whole, processed food. Fresh fruits and veggies, whole grains, lean proteins, and fermented foods like yogurt and kimchi can all help feed your gut and facilitate a healthy balance of bacteria in the process.

Include probiotic-rich foods: These are good bacteria which help in the gut. You add probiotic-rich foods or even supplements if you will, to counteract some of these nasty effects that maltodextrin does in your body.

Reduce Processed Food Items: Actually, strive to use fewer processed food products and those with long lists of ingredients. The greater the processing of a product, the higher the chances that it contains additives such as maltodextrin.

Let's discuss this issue with your doctor: perhaps you would need to talk to your doctor and explain whether, in fact, you have an issue with your gut, caused by digestive problems or other autoimmune disorders; discuss what you eat with your doctor or nutritionist and see if maltodextrin would impact the state of your gut.

Conclusion

The lesser danger that maltodextrin brings is on gut health. This food additive encourages the multiplication of bad bacteria in your gut, causes inflammation, and leads to leaky gut conditions- which can have devastating impacts on your digestive system in the long run. Never does one get a label with a digestive disorder due to maltodextrin but instead becomes a habitual consumption which generates chronic inflammation, which then goes as an input toward long-term health issues.

Moving on to the next chapter, we shall explore this inter-relationship between maltodextrin and inflammation: namely, how such an additive contributes to systemic inflammation and what that means in terms of chronic diseases like heart disease and cancer.

Chapter 7 : Maltodextrin and Inflammation: The Silent Threat

Inflammation is your body's response to injury or infection. It fights off the bad guys, helps with healing, and promotes the repair of tissues that have been damaged. Chronic inflammation is at the root of everything from autoimmune disorders to cardiovascular disease, cancer, and so much more. While many of us equate inflammation with obvious causes-like infections or injuries-your diet is one of the biggest fueling agents for-or component in the reduction of-inflammation. Perhaps the sneakiest dietary cause of inflammation, though, is maltodextrin-a food additive often found in processed foods.

This chapter will elaborate on how inflammation functions in chronic diseases, how maltodextrin triggers inflammatory reactions in you, and what is the reason for this underestimated ingredient to become the silent threat towards your long term health. By the end of this article, you should know everything about how maltodextrin can provoke inflammatory responses in your body.

Friend or Foe?

Inflammation is a double-edged sword. Acute inflammation is beneficial and protective: if you damage your skin, your immune system recognizes that it views a foreign invader and sends in white blood cells to the area in an attempt to control infection and limit damage. Redness, swelling, and heat in the area of injury are indicative that your immune system is doing its thing.

This is adaptive in the short term but pathologic when inflammation continues. Chronic inflammation raises the issue of forcing through time over months or years rather than resolving an acute problem. Such inflation leads to damage to healthy tissues and organs. Such low-level long-duration inflammation has thus been associated with chronic diseases like heart disease and diabetes, arthritis, and even neurodegenerative diseases like Alzheimer's. Diet is one of the most culprits of chronic inflammation, and some foods exert to trigger or provoke inflammatory responses. Any food containing maltodextrin falls into this category.

Maltodextrin and Why It's Essential to Induce Inflammation

Since maltodextrin, which is further discussed above, is a processed carbohydrate that is easily absorbed into blood with a high glycemic index, yet only induces immediate impact on blood sugar levels, it triggers other mechanisms to create inflammation in many other ways.

1. Control of the Gut Microbiome

In the previous chapter, it was also mentioned that maltodextrin can further disrupt the balance of bacteria in the gut by fostering the flourishing of the harmful pathogens, such as E. coli and Salmonella, while suppressing the helpful bacteria. It has been suggested to allow for the exacerbation of inflammation throughout the body.

Gut microbiome Controls the Immune System and Inflammation. In this instance, excessive activation of the immune system may result in overgrowth populations of pathogenic bacteria causing whole-body-wide massive inflammatory responses along with suppression of beneficial bacteria populations. Gut inflammation may be a chronic condition and is thought to be linked to irritable bowel syndrome through inflammatory diseases of the bowel leading to leaky gut syndrome but has resonations far beyond the abdominal space. Dysbiosis in the gut can also lead to systemic inflammation, which is defined as the result of inflammation throughout the whole body.

2. Effect on Blood Glucose and Insulin Sensitivity

A high glycemic index with maltodextrin leads to quick rises in blood sugar that cause the release of insulin. Continued spikes in the blood sugar level eventually result in resistance to insulin as the body would less be responsive to insulin and could no longer keep the blood sugar at a normal level. Insulin resistance goes hand in hand with chronic inflammation because high blood sugar is toxic to blood vessels, increases oxidative stress, and provides a stimulus for inflammatory activity.

Another condition that represents a prodrome to type 2 diabetes is insulin resistance; this is the disease of chronic inflammation. In fact, inflammation is now recognized as a major pathogenetic pathway for the initiation and acceleration of diabetes. It now appears that regular consumption of maltodextrin can drive the inflammatory process, thus potentiating metabolic disorder.

3. Direct activation of the immune system

Research showed that maltodextrin can directly stimulate the immune system, increasing pro-inflammatory cytokines-the small proteins that regulate inflammation. While these cytokines play important roles in the body's immune response, excessive production causes inflammation, damaging healthy cells and tissues.

For example, maltodextrin increases the production of several pro-inflammatory cytokines, including IL-6 and TNF-α. These cytokines are associated with chronic inflammation and several disorders, including rheumatoid arthritis, cardiovascular disease, and cancer. Increasing production of these cytokines increases the underlying level of chronic inflammation, which may ultimately impair health.

Chronic Inflammation and Disease

There is scientific literature by the mile citing chronic inflammation with diseases. We'll be speaking below about a few of the major diseases that can be characterized by chronic inflammation, and just how maltodextrin may play into the progression of such disorders.

1. Heart Disease

Atherosclerosis is associated with inflammation; in this condition, the fatty elements clog up the arteries and consequently raise the possibility of suffering from heart attacks and strokes. An increase in blood sugar levels by the intake of high GI foods such as maltodextrin, leads to a chain of reactions involving inflammation that will make the blood vessels more prone to damage from cholesterol elements to lay down plaques.

Over time, this chronic inflammation causes destruction of the artery walls and makes it easy to cause blood clots, leading to blockage of blood flowing into the heart or brain. Even though you might not have heart disease among your family members, repeated consumption of pro-inflammatory food intake, which includes foods rich in maltodextrin, makes you susceptible to cardiovascular diseases.

2. Obesity

Chronic inflammation and obesity are mutually interrelated. On one hand, obesity, most particularly visceral fat-the fat around the organs results in the unleashing of inflammatory cytokines that fuels the inflammation in various parts of the body. On the other side, inflammatory-related food tends to cause weight gain because it deranges metabolic function and enhances the storage of fats.

As we discussed, maltodextrin will contribute to blood sugar spikes and insulin resistance, which have become established as risks for weight gain and obesity. Such a process can lead to the long-term outcome of creating a vicious cycle whereby inflammation promotes fat storage, and the greater excess of fat will promote more inflammation.

3. Cancer

Chronic inflammation is another well-known risk factor for cancer. Inflammatory cytokines stimulate cell proliferation and suppress mechanisms whereby the body naturally destroys abnormal or damaged cells; such factors can therefore drive the growth of cancers. Long-term inflammation causes DNA damage, hence promoting the survival environment of cancer cells.

Although maltodextrin itself is not a direct carcinogen, its ability to induce inflammation creates conditions that seem to supposedly enhance the risk of cancer development. For example, higher risks of developing colorectal cancer are associated with inflammatory bowel diseases wherein gut inflammation is chronic. Responses induced by maltodextrin may condition and even worsen this risk.

4. Autoimmune Diseases

Autoimmune diseases are conditions in which the immune response attacks healthy tissues of the body, which leads to inflammation and tissue damage. Besides other forms of autoimmune diseases, chronic inflammation causes rheumatoid arthritis, lupus, multiple sclerosis, and psoriasis.

Other than that, maltodextrin may contribute to developing or worsening autoimmune diseases. It might also interfere with inflammation and gut health.

Hyperactivation of the gut alongside release of inflammatory cytokines leads to the autosensitization and initiation of autoimmune responses especially in those with predisposition to the diseases from a genetic standpoint.

How to Reduce Inflammation

Since maltodextrin may lead to chronic inflammation, its consumption should also be minimized along with inflammation in general. Here are some guidelines:

Have an Anti-Inflammatory Diet: Focus on whole foods naturally that have less inflammatory effects. These are leafy greens, fatty fish rich in omega-3 fatty acids, nuts, seeds, and antioxidant-rich fruits like berries. Avoid processed foods, especially maltodextrin and other additives.

Include Anti-Inflammatory Supplements: Turmeric contains curcumin; omega-3 fish oil, and ginger are also anti-inflammatory. Just make sure to include them in your daily routine and then know how you are neutralizing the inflammation process.

Cut Sugary Foods and Refined Carbohydrates from the Diet: Maltodextrin, like other refined carbohydrates, will raise blood sugar levels and lead to inflammation in the body. Be cautious of foods that are readymade, sugary food products, white bread, sugary snacks, etc.

Exercise: The best prevention against chronic inflammation is maintaining an active lifestyle. Exercise is one of the effective ways that keeps blood sugar levels in check, helps improve cardiovascular health, and creates an anti-inflammatory environment in the body.

Manage Stress: Chronic stress is one of the major causes of inflammation. Therefore, some people, using mindfulness, yoga, or deep breathing, can reduce inflammation and help achieve general well-being.

Consult a Doctor: If you are concerned about chronic inflammation or what it does to your body, take a visit to a health care provider who can point you in the right direction of what kind of diet and lifestyle changes will keep its risks at bay.

Conclusion

Perhaps one of the most insidious dangers of maltodextrin is its proinflammatory role. Working to damage your health in your gut, contributing to insulin resistance, and directly stimulating inflammatory responses, maltodextrin can fuel chronic inflammation that underlies most common and deadly diseases today. Limiting your intake of maltodextrin, while embracing an anti-inflammatory diet and lifestyle, can go a long way toward safeguarding your health and reducing your risk of disease caused by inflammation.

However, one thing we will look at in chapter two is how maltodextrin impacts the immune system and how it can utterly make your body's defenses lax and more vulnerable to diseases and chronic illness.

Chapter 8 : Maltodextrin and the Immune System: Breaking Down Your Body's Defence System

Your immunity system is your body's first line of defense against infections, pathogens, and at times abnormal cells, such as those that cause cancer. The healthy functioning of the immune system is identified by destroying invading pathogens while keeping healthy tissues intact; indeed, some foods and additives, such as maltodextrin, may disrupt this sensitive system and leave it more open to infection, diseases, and autoimmune disorders.

How Maltodextrin Disrupts Immune Function

These mechanisms tend to explain how maltodextrin suppresses the immune system. From encouraging proliferation of pathogenic bacteria to exacerbating inflammation, a perfect storm is created that attacks your body's defenses over time.

1. Gut Health and Immune Function: A Delicate Balance

We discussed in previous chapters how gut health is associated with immune function. Indeed, it is estimated that about 70% of the immune cells live within the gut, and thus it is a very important player in terms of immune reactions. Healthy gut microbiomes will help regulate immune response;

this means that the immune system will have an appropriate reaction towards harmful invaders but will take precautionary measures to avoid overreaction.

This disrupts the flora balance since it supports the proliferation of harmful bacteria, such as E. coli, and suppresses beneficial bacteria, for example Lactobacillus reuteri. Dysbiosis destroys the immunity regulation capacity within the gut by proliferating pathogenic bacteria that cause inappropriate immune responses in relation to chronic inflammation within the body as well as failure of its defense mechanism against infections.

Dysbiosis also disrupts the gut barrier, which is a mechanical barrier that prevents pathogens from entering the bloodstream. When weakened, one develops something called "leaky gut," which means pathogens, toxins, and undigested food particles leak into the bloodstream. This can easily overburden the immune system, forcing it to work harder in neutralizing these invaders, and will oftentimes lead to chronic inflammation.

2. Facilitating Pathogenic Bacterial Growth

One study also showed that maltodextrin may increase the biofilm formation of Salmonella within the intestinal tract, thus increasing the chance of infection; the immunocompromised and chronic diseases put anyone in a special at-risk group because their immune system would not clear up infections caused by such bacteria.

In addition, the presence of harmful bacteria such as E. coli in the gut leads to widespread inflammation that further compromises the immune response. Chronic inflammation weakens the immune response of an individual to react against new pathogens, leaving the individual more vulnerable to infections, illnesses, and chronic diseases.

3. Suppression of Beneficial Bacteria

The positive effect is stimulating unwanted bacteria in the gut; on the other hand, it restricts normal beneficial bacteria. The two types of beneficial bacteria are Lactobacillus and Bifidobacterium. These types of bacteria aid greatly in immune activity by controlling the rate at which certain immune cells are produced, keeping the integrity of the gut wall and preventing unwanted bacteria from controlling the gut.

Maltodextrin not only decreases the number of good bacteria but weakens the body's natural defense mechanisms, making it less competent to fight off infections. Moreover, such inhibition of good bacteria might lead to a possible autoimmune reaction, in which the body attacks its own tissues mistakenly.

4. Induction of Inflammatory Responses

As explained in Chapter 6, maltodextrin acts as a pro-inflammatory cytokines' activator—those proteins responsible for regulating the body's immune response. Even though, without a doubt, these cytokines are important for fighting infections, their overproduction might lead to chronic inflammation and then cause irreparable damages to tissues and organs while weakening the immunity by flooding it with continuous threats.

In fact, studies have shown that maltodextrin may induce the activity of certain cytokines, such as IL-6 and TNF-α, which are associated with chronic inflammation and immunological dysfunction. Such a chronic phase of inflammation slowly impairs the ability of the immune system to recognize and eliminate newly-emerging pathogens and tumor cells.

5. Increased Vulnerability to Autoimmune Diseases

The immune system needs to recognize what's foreign and to distinguish it from healthy cells of the body. Once this fails, because of chronic inflammation and gut dysbiosis as another example, it can begin to attack the body's own tissues, leading to autoimmune diseases.

After inducing gut permeability and inflammation, the immune system starts responding to healthy tissues as pathogens, which may cause rheumatoid arthritis, lupus, and multiple sclerosis. The body gets an adverse reaction against its own organs and tissues as a result of this malfunctioning of the immune system.

6. Immune Response to Pathogens

Infection is, therefore, considered a direct test of the efficacy of the immune system in responding to pathogens. When the immune system cannot fight infections promptly because of such factors as poor gut health and chronic inflammation, the body is more susceptible to acute and chronic conditions.

For example, an immunocompromised individual is likely more vulnerable to infections which are caused by pathogenic bacteria such as E. coli and Salmonella. Both E. coli and Salmonella will grow in the presence of maltodextrin. For the vulnerably Immunocompromised members of society, like the elderly and chronically ill patients, this increased susceptibility is critically important.

Even more, an immunity system malice can be unable to curb viral infections. Maltodextrin induced chronic low-grade inflammation continues to hinder the immune system from properly reacting against viruses like the flu or even colds. Due to frequent infections, their immunity can be further weakened, therefore generating a vicious cycle of illnesses and unhealthy living.

How To Protect Your Immune System

The good news, however, is that you can take measures that protect your immune system and minimize the damage maltodextrin does to your body. A healthy diet and proper lifestyle can help support immune function, thus reducing infections and chronic diseases.

Practical tips:

Minimize Your Intake of Processed Food: It is also best to totally avoid the foods that contain maltodextrin if you can. Actually, one simple way to avoid excessive exposure to this ingredient is to minimize your intake of processed food. Overall, even though it is now clear that maltodextrin is generally not harmful to health, food experts would advise people to stick to nutrient-dense whole foods that contribute to a healthy immune system, such as fruits, vegetables, whole grains, and lean proteins.

Consume probiotic: Probiotic foods such as yoghurt, kefir, sauerkraut, and kimchi that are rich in live microorganisms and, therefore, facilitate healthy gut bacteria and immune systems.

Increase Anti-Inflammatory Foods: Food intake rich in omega-3 fatty acids, such as salmon, walnuts, and flaxseeds, can reduce inflammation, supporting the immune system. Foods that are high in antioxidants, such as berries, leafy greens, and turmeric, may mediate oxidative stress and inflammation.

Prioritize sleep and stress management: Chronic stress and lack of sleep will weaken the immune system in order to fight infections. Prioritize good sleep hygiene and stress-reduction techniques such as meditation, yoga, or deep breathing to help support your immune system.

Consult a Healthcare Provider: Should you become more concerned with the health of your immune system, and especially if you have a history of autoimmune diseases or infections, go see a healthcare provider. They will guide you on how to adjust your dietary and lifestyle choices to strengthen your immune system.

Conclusion:

That is because the most dangerous effects of maltodextrin can undermine your immune system. It gives way to unhealthy growth in bacteria, and it's a source of chronic inflammation, which makes your natural defensive mechanism weaker and more susceptible to infections and autoimmune disorders. All this requires some adjustments either to lessen its consumption in your diet or to keep healthy lifestyle and dietary habits so that your health is protected, and the immune system remains robust.

The association of maltodextrin with mental health will thus be a subject of the next chapter, discussing how, with regards to its impact on mood and cognition, it might have a role in the etiology of neurological disorders.

Chapter 9 : Maltodextrin and Psychiatric Illnesses

The connection between what you eat and how you feel runs far more profoundly than might be initially obvious. While most know that diet affects physical well-being, few comprehend the depth with which food selections affect mental health. Like any other organ, the brain is a product of what it is fed-or, rather, a product of what it is not fed. Scientific research published recently indicates that some food additives, such as maltodextrin, can negatively impact mood and thought processes, and even foster the creation of mental illness.

Now, in this chapter, we look at the unsuspected nexus between maltodextrin and mental health. We will critically examine how a food additive so commonly used can influence brain functioning, mood stability, and cognitive processes. We shall also review the latest literature about a link between maltodextrin and anxiety, depression, and neurodegenerative disorders including Alzheimer's. You will take the very first steps to protect your mental well-being based on new knowledge about these connections.

The Brain-Gut Connection

The brain-gut connection is a prerequisite to understanding the impact maltodextrin has on mental health. The gut and the brain are in a close communication network of neurons, hormones, and neurotransmitters termed the gut-brain axis. The gut-brain axis plays an important role in mood regulation, cognition, and mental wellbeing.

A key player in this system is the gut microbiome, a community of bacteria and other microbes found in the digestive tract. These microbes produce neurotransmitters -serotonin and dopamine being two examples- that help us manage our moods and emotions. As an interesting aside, most of the body's serotonin-the neurotransmitter that keeps our moods in check-is made in the gut. Because of these processed foods and additives-maltodextrin, for example-there are times that the intestine gets thrown out of kilter. This sensitive network has its communications disturbed.

1. Maltodextrin Effects on Gut Microbiome

Maltodextrin upsets the balance of the gut microbiome by boosting maladaptive populations, such as the proliferation of bad bacteria in the gut and a reduction of the population of beneficial strains, like Lactobacillus and Bifidobacterium. The shift in balance in the gut microbiota is known as dysbiosis and then contributes to widespread consequences in the brain, which include mood disorders, including anxiety and depression.

A balanced gut microbiome assists in the regulation of inflammation, neurotransmitter production, and the body's stress response-all factors that impact mental health. However, when there is a state of dysbiosis, the levels of neurotransmitters in the brain which are good for stabilizing mood such as serotonin and GABA decrease while pro-inflammatory molecules increase. This combination produces a biochemical environment likely to induce those feelings of anxiety, depression, and mood swings.

2. Inflammation and the Brain

However, another potential way maltodextrin affects mental health is by inflammation. As discussed in Chapter 6, we know that maltodextrin triggers the expression of pro-inflammatory cytokines, thus resulting in chronic low-grade inflammation. It has been found just recently that there is a strong link between chronic inflammation and diseases in the mental health category, such as depression, anxiety, and even cognitive impairment.

The inflammation of the brain damages the neurons and disrupts the normal functioning of the brain by interfering with neurotransmitter production. The presence of mental health symptoms that result from this inflammation includes fatigue, mood disturbances, and cognitive impairments. Research studies have shown that patients suffering from depression present high levels of inflammatory markers in their bloodstream; this leads scientists to believe that eliminating or reducing inflammation may help alleviate depressive symptoms.

3. The Role of Blood Sugar and Insulin Resistance in Mood Disorders

Rapid absorption and digestion of maltodextrin can also affect mental status because its consumption encourages unstable blood sugar. The moment you consume foods containing maltodextrin, your blood sugar will shoot up as fast as it will drop afterwards. This cycle can lead to irritability, fatigue, and brain fogginess - common symptoms that impact mood and cognitive function.

Over time, repeated blood sugar surges cause the body's cells to become unresponsive to insulin. Insulin resistance has been linked to an increased risk of mood disorders. It worsens both depression and anxiety. Stable blood sugar levels allow the brain to function at its full potential, but frequent flux deafferented the brain from both mood and cognition regulation.

4. Leaky Gut and the Blood-Brain Barrier

Similarly, since maltodextrin could jeopardize the integrity of the intestinal wall, thus causing leaky gut syndrome, the blood-brain barrier may also be impaired. This is a cell layer that protects harmful substances in the blood from reaching the brain. Once this protective layer is breached, the toxic and inflammatory molecules and pathogens start penetrating into the brain, thereby setting off inflammation and neurodegeneration.

A leaky blood-brain barrier has been linked to numerous mental health disorders, such as depression, anxiety, and Alzheimer's disease. In that sense, maltodextrin may be linked to having a chance of dysfunction on the blood-brain barrier that may lead to cognitive and emotional symptoms.

Maltodextrin and Psychosis

Since the connection between the brain and the gut, inflammation, and blood sugar instability, let us take a closer look at the specific mental health conditions maltodextrin could be linked with.

1. Depression

A multifactorial mental disorder involving genetic, environmental, and lifestyle factors, depression has lately been linked to diet and gut health. Inflammation, dysbiosis, blood sugar level fluctuations, and many more aspects are associated with the consumption of maltodextrin in the development of depression, all of which are pivotal factors.

It will be noted that with improved inflammation and a bad gut, the production of neurotransmitter level decreases, which can lead to depression-like symptoms. People who are suffering with depression usually have more inflammatory biomarkers, and anti-inflammatory treatment also improves the symptoms of depression.

Besides, emerging research indicates that insulin resistance, which maltodextrin enhances, makes a person more vulnerable to depression. A particular study suggested that depressed patients are mostly those with insulin resistance. This indicates that stable sugar in the blood should be maintained for good mental health.

2. Anxiety

Similar to depression, there is also a strong relationship between anxiety and inflammation, gut health, and control of blood sugar. Studies have shown that people with anxiety disorders are often affected by an imbalance in the gut microbiome, and improvement in gut health relieves the symptoms of anxiety.

Maltodextrin disrupts gut dysbiosis and inflammation, which induces anxiety through an interruption of the gut-brain axis. If good bacteria are repressed and bad ones proliferate, synthesis of neurotransmitters related to mood regulation and anxiety will be impaired, such as GABA. This only makes it worse how well the brain can cope with stress and anxiety.

This instability in blood sugar levels brought about by rapid absorption in maltodextrin can also cause anxiety symptoms. This is because whenever the body experiences a drastic drop in blood sugar due to a sudden rise, stress hormones such as cortisol and adrenaline are released, which boosts feelings of anxiety and nervousness and irritability.

3. Decline in Cognitive Ability and Alzheimer's Disease

More recent studies come to the limelight that increasingly suggest dietary factors drive cognitive health and subsequent risks in dementia from neurodegenerative conditions like Alzheimer's. Specifically, these losses are driven by the two major mechanisms, namely inflammation and insulin resistance, which have been associated with maltodextrin intake.

Chronic inflammation within the brain can cause neurons to degenerate and even lead to impaired cognitive abilities which might lead to memory loss, confusion, and difficulties in concentrating. The product is also thought to be implicated in the formation of amyloid plaques, abnormal deposits in the brain that are associated with Alzheimer's disease.

These are augmented by other risk factors, such as insulin resistance, which is associated with cognitive decline. Some researchers have even said that Alzheimer's disease should be referred to as "type 3 diabetes" due to the close association of its etiopathogeny with insulin resistance and neurodegeneration. When a part of the body becomes less responsive to insulin, a corresponding reduced use of glucose for energy subsequently occurs, which in turn causes impairment in cognition.

Maltodextrin may cause inflammation and insulin resistance, potentially impairing the development of neurodegenerative diseases and cognitive decline. Reducing your maltodextrin intake and following a brain-healthy diet will help prevent deterioration in your mental abilities with advancing age.

Protecting Your Psychological Health

Though maltodextrin's impact on your psychological well-being is scary, there are some ways through which you can safeguard your brain and your mental health. Here are several strategies that you may look into:

Eat for Your Mental Health: Focus on whole foods that will nourish the brain and stabilize mood. Make sure to get good amounts of omega-3-rich food sources such as fatty fish, flaxseeds, and walnuts. In addition, add plenty of antioxidant-rich fruits and vegetables to your diet. It would do well to eliminate foods that are processed, maltodextrin, and other additives that impair gut health and have a sense of inflammation.

Gut Health: Establish a healthy gut microbiome - critically important to mental health. Focus on probiotic-rich foods like yogurt, kefir, and sauerkraut, which will help to replenish friendly bacteria. The prebiotic fibers in foods such as garlic, onions, and bananas feed these bacteria.

Control Blood Sugar: Maintain the blood sugar at a steady point so that emotions are kept under control and in a healthy condition. Avoid foods that cause the spikes of blood sugar, especially those foods highly prepared with refined carbohydrates and sugars. Eat whole grains, lean proteins, and healthy fats to release slow energy.

Reduces Inflammation: An anti-inflammatory diet can certainly be a positive powerful protector to your body and mind. There are foods such as turmeric, leafy greens, berries, and fatty fish, that are mighty anti-inflammatory agents which help promote brain function while reducing the risk of mood disorders.

Practice mindfulness and stress management: Chronic stress may predispose the impact of maltodextrin on mental health. Use yoga, meditation, or deep breathing exercises among the myriad of mindfulness exercises to reduce and manage the effects of stress on your emotional well-being.

Keeping Active: Physically active lives, not only helps reduce inflammation and build brain health but also boosts moods and cognitive functions. It increases the production of endorphins and neurotransmitters which enhance feelings of wellbeing and help in regulating mood. Do at least 150 minutes a week of moderate aerobic activity, strength training exercises to maximize mental and physical health benefits.

Sleep Adequately: Good quality of sleep is the requirement for good mental health and cognitive performance. Adults should sleep for 7-9 hours daily to ensure that the brain is recharged, memories consolidated, and the mood regulated. Establish a bedtime routine that helps you relax and limits your exposure to all kinds of screens before bedtime.

Consult a healthcare professional, such as a mental health professional or registered dietitian, if you have mood disorders, cognitive decline, or any other mental health issues. They will be able to craft a plan for your particular needs, taking into account the patterns of your dietary habits and lifestyle practices.

Conclusion

The relationship of maltodextrin to mental health is somewhat complex, driven through interplay between dietary intake, gut health, inflammation, and brain function. A breakdown in the balance of this gut microbiome due to maltodextrin and the induction of inflammatory responses can drive mood disorders, anxiety, cognitive decline, and neurodegenerative diseases.

Taking proactive steps in trying to reduce your intake of maltodextrin and doing everything possible through nutrition, proper stress management, and changing one's lifestyle can help preserve emotional well-being. What you eat today might be what haunts you mentally in the future. So, eat to achieve a balanced diet by only eating whole, nutrient-rich foods.

The next chapter on maltodextrin discusses the regulatory environment under which maltodextrin operates, including its classification, labeling, and other information to be provided to the consumer. Such education will empower you to make better choices for your health through your food.

Chapter 10 : The Regulatory Landscape of Maltodextrin

As a consumer, awareness of the regulatory framework surrounding food additives like maltodextrin can be very useful in more informed dietary choices. Food additives such as maltodextrin are regulated by various agencies, and the regulations between countries can be significantly different. This chapter explains how maltodextrin is classified, the safety assessments made by the regulatory bodies, and its impact on consumers with regard to labeling and transparency related to food and food industry operations.

1. What is Maltodextrin?

Perhaps a good place to start would be to define exactly what maltodextrin is. Maltodextrin is a carbohydrate extracted from starch. It is most commonly produced from corn, rice, or potato starch. It's mostly a white powder that is easily soluble in water, making it a popular ingredient in various processed foods. Maltodextrin often serves as a thickener, filler, or sweetener for products like snack bars and chips, sauces, salad dressings, and even dietary supplements.

Although widely used, many consumers do not know if it exists in their food supply, mainly because it often hides under generic labeling. That brings us to the regulatory environment.

2. Regulatory Agencies and Safety Assessments

In the United States, maltodextrin is one of the food additives that the FDA oversees for safety and regulatory controls. The FDA demands that a thorough safety assessment be done on any food additive before it will be approved for use in food products. Also, testing for the additive is relatively broad in scope, taking into account possible health risks as well as a potential for long-term effects.

Maltodextrin is "Generally Recognized as Safe" (GRAS) by the FDA. That is, experts widely agree that this ingredient is safe for consumption under its intended conditions of use. Even though it may have been declared GRAS, this does not necessarily mean that it poses no health threats; it just means that it is generally accepted as safe by scientific consensus.

EFSA (European Food Safety Authority) also evaluates food additives and their safety in the European Union. EFSA conducted the same risk assessment and established that maltodextrin is safe for consumption at certain quantities. They still propose tracking the daily intake to prevent overconsumption of this additive, mainly because it is used extensively in processed foods.

3. Labeling Practices and Transparency

One of the most significant issues related to maltodextrin is its labeling in food items. Consumers may not know they have maltodextrin unless they read the ingredient list at the back of the package. Ingredient descriptions are often just referred to as "maltodextrin," without indicating the possible source or health effects. This can be quite confusing for consumers and make it difficult to judge for them.

The other issue is that there is no regulation in the United States that mandates that food manufacturers would be required to declare the source of maltodextrin on product labels. The permitted ingredients are revealed on the packaging of any product, but there is no official declaration of what maltodextrin is derived from, for instance whether it's made from corn, rice, or potato. That might be a problem when consumers who are particular regarding dietary restrictions or allergies were trying to pinpoint where their maltodextrin was coming from because some types of maltodextrin are produced from GMOs.

But in a way, the European Union is stricter in its labeling laws, especially on labeling food additives and its source. For example, if maltodextrin is a GMO byproduct, this must be indicated in the label. This level of transparency places a consumer in a better position to make decisions about what they buy.

4. Consumer Advocacy and Education

It is, however, the consumer organizations and groups that should be able to pressure society into more truthfulness in labeling. Many of the consumer groups advocate for stricter regulations about food additives. Consumer groups shall also educate themselves on what they eat.

Consumers need to be aware of what's in the ingredient label and know which products contain maltodextrin, especially those tagged as "healthy" and "natural." Knowing what maltodextrin does, particularly in huge amounts, will lead consumers into more wholesome decisions.

5. Shopping at the Store: What's the Consumer to Do?

As you are shopping at the store and finding items that are maltodextrin-free, here are some real-life guidelines:

Read Labels: Make a conscious look at maltodextrin in an ingredient list of processed foods. Be on the lookout for alternatives without maltodextrin and as much whole food as possible without added ingredients.

Eat More Whole Foods: Buy more whole, unprocessed foods like fruits, vegetables, whole grains, lean proteins, and healthy fats. Generally, whole, unprocessed foods contain no maltodextrin.

Learn About Better Brands: Know the brand that is transparent and adds minimal additives to labels. Most of the companies today keep focusing on clean labels and not using ingredients which are controversial.

Ask Questions: If unsure, ask the store employees or the manufacturer to provide the details.

Make Your Own: Sauce preparation, snack, meal preparations are very easy. This way, you are in charge of the ingredients and avoid maltodextrin altogether.

6. The Future of Food Additives and Consumer Protection

Public awareness grows by leaps and bounds, and thus the demand for transparency regarding food ingredients and ever-stricter regulation on the part of the food industry grows in crescendo. Consumers grow ever more active as health promoters and advocates for cleaner food options.

Some regulatory agencies are already responding to this growing demand. For example, the FDA recently showed willingness to review the safety of every food additive if new information arrives about it. This could mean more stringent regulations for maltodextrin and other additives in the future.

Also, as more consumers are looking for healthier choices, the producers would be prompted to reformulate the products and eliminate the unnecessary additives present in the products. This is already happening, among other factors that explain the reason why the organic and clean-label products are gaining tremendous popularity-they generally avoid synthetic ingredients and prefer wholesome ingredients.

Conclusion

It is essential knowledge for people who want to make healthy food choices. While maltodextrin is declared safe by regulatory offices, it pops up a lot in processed food, and it may serve as a trigger for health hazards. With considerable diligence in reading labels, advocating transparency, and whole foods, such an intake of maltodextrin can be curtailed, and your health preserved.

In the next chapter, I will offer some very practical suggestions for reducing the maltodextrin in your diet: tips on cooking, shopping, and meal planning. "Knowledge is power" might be a good way to phrase that.

Chapter 11 : Strategies To Reduce The Intake of Maltodextrin In Your Diet

Due to the growing awareness of health risks caused by the additive maltodextrin, most consumers begin seeking efficient ways to minimize or eliminate the presence of this additive in their food. In this chapter, we address some actionable steps or ways to minimize intake of maltodextrin: cooking tips, shopping guides, and meal planning suggestions. Engaging with these strategies in everyday life gives you control over your food choices and therefore better health.

1. Be Aware of Its Sources

The first step in controlling maltodextrin in your diet is to be able to determine the most common sources of its presence in food and other edible products. Maltodextrin, as an additive, can be found in any of the following processed food:

i) Thickener-used in sauces, dressings, and gravies

ii) Filling agent-used in a snack bar, powdered drink mix, meal replacement

iii) Sweetener-used in sugar-free or reduced-calorie products

iv) Preservative-may be added to extend product shelf life.

v) Knowing what most of these uses of maltodextrin are would help to read it while finding products.

2. Be Careful to Read Ingredient Labels

To steer clear of maltodextrin, then reading ingredient labels carefully is of utmost importance. Some of the things on which you should look out while on a shopping spree include the following:

Ingredient List: You should at all times be looking for maltodextrin on the ingredient list. When maltodextrin is available, then it becomes necessary to look elsewhere for a product that doesn't contain this additive.

Common Interchangeable Terms: Keep in mind that maltodextrin can be masked under other terms, and this is very true in the case of the product being sugar-laden and is labelled as "healthy" or "natural." Common terms to look out for are "corn syrup solids" or "dextrin."

Allergen Information: If you have allergies or special dietary needs, also look for labelling regarding potential allergens concerning the source of maltodextrin.

3. Eat Whole, Unprocessed Foods

Some of the best ways to reduce the consumption of maltodextrin would be through ensuring that one takes a diet rich in whole, unprocessed foods. For some quick incorporation of more whole foods into your diet, try these:

Fresh Produce: Pack the shopping cart with fruits and vegetables for optimal nutrient-rich foods that are naturally additive-free.

Whole Grains: Replace the grain products containing maltodextrin as refinement with whole grains such as quinoa, brown rice, oats, and whole wheat.

Lean protein: Use fresh, whole or minimally processed meats, poultry, fish, eggs, and legumes and tofu as sources of lean proteins.

Healthy fats: Use healthy fats like avocados, nuts, seeds, and pure olive oil that have no added preservatives.

With this strategy, you will focus on whole foods, ensuring the least likelihood of having maltodextrin added to your diet and more nutrients.

4. Cook at Home

It encompasses taking full control of ingredients used when preparing your meals while cooking at home. This is a wonderful strategy to reduce your maltodextrin intake. Here are some cooking tips:

Cook Sauces and Dressings: Prepare your sauces and dressings from scratch instead of buying the pre-packaged kinds found in stores that may contain maltodextrin. Some simple recipes for tomato sauce, vinaigrettes, and marinades can be prepared using fresh ingredients.

Snack Wisely: Mostly, packaged snacks contain maltodextrin. Snack with whole ingredients- nuts, seeds, and dried fruits in trail mix or simply make your own popcorn and season it with herbs and spices.

Cook Meals in Batches: Meal prepping can assist you in planning your meals for the whole week and ensure that you have control over what ends up in each dish. Cook big portions of grains, proteins, and vegetables that you can mix and match at different times of the week, cutting your reliance on processed foods. 5. Look for Healthier Alternatives

Where you find packaged products that contain Maltodextrin, seek out a healthier alternative. Some options include:

Ration Bars: Choose whole food bars, such as those with nuts, seeds, and dried fruits. Avoid them if maltodextrin is listed as an ingredient.

Drink Mixes: If you need a drink mix, choose an unsweetened powdered mix or flavored water. Avoid them if maltodextrin is listed as an ingredient.

Pouch or Packaged Meals: Opt for frozen or pre-cooked meals that make the most of wholesome ingredients. Avoid additives like maltodextrin.

6. Become Informed on Brands

Find brands that focus on clean, transparent ingredients. Many today are dedicated to having few additives and clearly labeling. On the go:

Check the company's website: Most websites have a long list of ingredients as well as information about the sourcing practices. Sometimes this helps you make a decision about which ones fit your needs regarding health goals.

Look for Certifications: Look at products that have a certification, like whether they are organic or non-GMO. Many times, the process of getting certified means that there are no artificial additives in them.

7. Harness the Power of Technology

In this contemporary technological world, apps and websites can alert customers to what to choose to make the very best healthy food choices. These are useful in making the best decisions of what one should consume:

Ingredient Scanning Apps: These applications allow you to scan barcodes of products to access information directly about the ingredients with potential allergens and additives like maltodextrin.

Nutrition Trackers: You may be able to track overall intake of additives using nutrition tracking apps as you monitor other decisions.

8. Interacting with Community Resources

Engage in local health organizations or online forums regarding healthy food and nutrition. Most of these resources provide access to knowledge, recipes, and support for reducing additives in food. Some good suggestions are:

Cooking Classes: Join local cooking classes that teach how to prepare whole food. Such classes can help you be a stronger cook but also will give inspiration for new recipes.

Health Seminars: Attend seminars or workshops which touch on nutrition and awareness in ingredients. Such an event often provides insightful information from an expert source, as well as networks of like-minded people to interact with.

Conclusion

It takes education and concerted effort to reduce the amount of maltodextrin in one's diet. Knowing where it is most frequently consumed comes next, or rather what it is most typically found in, what foods. It guides one in deciphering additives on labels; it educates individuals towards whole foods and consumption is definitely achievable through community resources.

The book continues into personal experiences and personal testimonies from individuals who changed their diet in avoiding maltodextrin, along with the benefits they received as an approach to health and well-being. First-hand accounts can be inspirational for you starting your journey to better eating.

Chapter 12 : Personal Stories and Testimonials: Turning Lives Around By Avoiding Maltodextrin

As we go through the remainder of the journey of hidden perils of maltodextrin, we will need to keep in mind how the real-life changes in diet may be playing out for an individual's health and wellness. To share some real-life stories and testimonies, in this chapter, I will walk you through the experiences of people who have specifically reduced or even quit the intake of maltodextrin in their diet. The more precious experiences of these people illustrate benefits of this choice, representing insights to the possibility of transformation through mindful eating as an intervention.

1. Sarah's Road from Slumber to Energy Case study: Sarah, a 34-year-old mother of two, embarked on a journey after suffering from chronic fatigue and digestive problems. Sarah ate what seemed a healthy diet, but she often relied on plenty of so-called convenience foods containing maltodextrin. A nutritionist counseled her on the possible effects of additives like maltodextrin on her body.

"I was really shocked to learn how many of the snacks and meals I relied on had maltodextrin in them," Sarah said. "Once I started reading labels, I found out it was everywhere! I decided it was time to make a change."

For cooking healthier meals for their family, Sarah dedicated herself to taking on the extra work and keeping her diets whole. According to her, after quitting the processed snack and meal habit, she felt more energetic and relieved her discomfort about digestive problems.

"Within a few weeks, I felt more energetic than I had for years. My digestion improved and I even lost a few pounds without trying!", she said, stressing how her general health and vitality had drastically improved since she made alterations in diet.

2. Mark's battle with anxiety

Mark K Now, Mark is a 28-year-old graphic designer who has suffered with anxiety most of his adult life. All too often, he would pop open a bag of chips, a can of soda or an energy drink-most of which held maltodextrin. He didn't think it had anything to do with the bouts of anxiety, but a discussion with a friend changed his perception.

"My friend was saying that some additives, like maltodextrin, can affect mood and anxiety levels. I decided to dig deeper to learn more and found that there were indeed a couple of studies on how diet impacts mental health," Mark said.

Mark felt anxiety reduction when he stopped the foods that contained maltodextrin and switched primarily to fruits, green leafy vegetables, lean proteins, and whole grains.

I began to become calmer and less anxious, too, he said. It is amazing how much food can impact your mood. Today I am more watchful with regards to what I eat and feel a thousand times better.

3. Jessica's Discovery

Jessica is a health coach with 45 years. For years, she has been helping clients reach their wellness objectives. She recently realized that scrutinizing her diet was essential only after she faced her health challenges. In pursuing healthier living, Jessica had consumed maltodextrin-containing protein powders and meal replacement shakes.

"After using those products for a few months, I started noticing unexplained weight gain and extreme tiredness," Jessica explained. "I felt slow, and my skin was full of breakouts, so I started checking out the ingredients, and that is when I found maltodextrin."

She decided to replace processed foods with whole foods and opted for natural protein sources like legumes, nuts, and seeds. At the end of this, she found that she not only lost the extra weight but her energy increased to a phenomenal height, and her skin cleared.

At Whole Foods "This was probably the most enlightening (for me). Jessica says, "Then I was like – Man… I feel so much better without that crap in my life!! So I should teach my clients why they need to know at least a little bit of what is in their food..

4. Tom's Journey with Gut Health

Tom, 52; Engineer He had a GI disorder for years that affected his quality of life. And it was not until Tom self-referred to a gastroenterologist years later that he learned making dietary changes would cure him. The white layer remained in Ryan's intestines, and Tom knew what maltodextrin additives did to the gut.

Tom says, "No clue what I was ingesting and in all probability hurting me. When I slightly modified the way I started eating - focusing more on real food and using a slight awareness of what I was eating to prevent processed poison - things just blew up big time…

He ramped up his fiber and probiotic consumption, mainly in the interest of digestive health, and also began to prepare all his meals instead of taking maltodextrin-laden meal replacements. Digestive problems slowly subsided over time.

"Feels like I got my life back," he said. Not having to worry about swallowing while eating is a gift. That, combined with my diet, should make everyone in the state reconsider their diets.

5. Community Impact: Starting the Conversation

Here are the stories of Sarah, Mark, Jessica, and Tom, which show a great deal of difference that knowledge about food makes for individuals. Their personal evolutions also help fuel healthy dialogue about our culture and why nutrition and ingredient consciousness are important.

They took conversations about food additives and health and wellness through friends, family, social media, etc. as they began to hear good things from the few people that had already kicked here in town. Others motivated their peers to get a bit more serious about eating as they did, adding more pieces to the building wave of better habits.

6. Building Support Group

As can be evident from each of these anecdotes, one major take-away is the importance of having a support system. Stories can uplift and inspire others through their healing journey. Maybe you were using online forums, local health groups, or just having random conversations with friends and family members. But, most importantly is the aid and motivation we can receive from someone else.

Creating a Support System

Scope out Facebook: join social media groups revolving around health and fitness. They could offer healthy tips or recipes, or ways to encourage each other.

Launch a Meetup: Forming a local group that meets up to talk about and exchange healthy meal plans is another great idea.

Enroll at Workshops and Classes: Look for some opportunities in your area that focuses on nutrition education, cooking classes or healthy life. The interplay with like-minded kind of people strengthens the progressions.

Conclusion

It is controversial because it relates to the physiological consequences of dietary changes and the effect on health and mortality. In fact, the stories of other life-changers like Sarah, Mark and Jessica and Tom might just as easily show how their MAL-freeness turned into some improvements in quality of life.

From there reflect on their experiences, and how you can relate those principles to your life. It also means that everyone can tweak their diet a little and gain improvements in the way they feel, just maybe hearing your story will give some people inspiration to do so.

The next chapter looks at how awareness and education are great ways to combat artificial food additives, particularly in regards to an individual or community war on unhealthy eating habits, while working with transparency in the industry.

Chapter 13 : Education And Awareness Towards Food Additives Role

As we consider maltodextrin and its possible health effects, it's high time to promote education and awareness in overcoming the hurdles created by food additives. We will present within this chapter how, together with individuals and communities, their efforts may come into play for better habits of consumption, campaigns for more transparency in food labeling, and the encouragement of an ethos of enlightened nutrition choice.

1. The Importance of Education

Education is the basis of enlightened nutritional decisions. Understanding what is in your food-what maltodextrin is, for example-is the first step in taking control of one's health and well-being. Food education includes the following key items:

Ingredient Literacy: Basic understanding of ingredients in foods-including where they come from, what they do, and what their potential health implications may be-is vital. It will empower customers with better choices and make them think about what they're eating.

Nutrition Basics: Understanding basic nutrition principles, including macronutrients (carbohydrates, proteins, fats) and micronutrients (vitamins and minerals), helps individuals recognize the importance of a balanced diet rich in whole foods.

Health Awareness: Increased awareness of the potential health risks associated with processed foods and additives can motivate individuals to seek healthier alternatives.

2. Community Initiatives: Building Awareness Together

Communities are at the forefront of education on food additives as well as healthy dietary choice. Here are some ways that communities can act together:

Hold workshops and seminars: Organizing training talks on how nutrition, food labeling, and impacts of additives could be discussed might provide an insight into the community. Such events might be very informative and useful in telling people about a healthier way to eat.

School Programs: Nutrition education in schools will provide children with healthy eating habits. Food labeling, cooking, and informed choice education could create a generation of health-conscious individuals.

Health Fairs and Events: Organizing community-based health fairs with the involvement of local business and organizations promoting healthy food, cooking demonstrations, and discussion on food additives will get people to talk about nutrition.

3. Advocacy for Clear Labeling

Advocacy is one of the tools that can help in ensuring transparency of food labeling. Consumers may unite to demand the clear label of foods so that manufacturers label their products clearly and accurately. Advocacy strategies include:

Call Officials: Encourage the community to call local elected officials and let them know how labeling practices of foods must change. This should make further tough regulations in regards to additives of food and allow for more transparent labeling.

Petition Signatures: Participate or initiate a petition that focuses on clearer labeling of foods and a restriction of objectionable additives can increase consumers' voices and get regulatory action taken.

Creating Social Media Campaigns: Use social media avenues to disseminate information about maltodextrin, other food additives, and the need for clarity. This would help achieve a broad outreach for a movement toward healthier foods .

4. Empowerment of Consumers

Consumers, as they are better informed about the foods they consume, can take proactive measures to safeguard themselves.

Empowering Strategies for Consumers:

Learn and Educate Oneself and Others: Be informed about the new scientific research on food additives, nutrition, and healthy eating. Based on that knowledge, inform people around you, especially family and friends, to sway choices at the grassroots level.

Communitary Gardens: Participate in a community garden to help get closer to one's food and promote growing fruits and vegetables for cooking. In the process of growing it, one will attain further nutrition and production knowledge.

Cooking Classes: Engage, or host cooking classes on healthy preparation of whole foods. Knowing that food can be prepared both healthily and freshly will give people the confidence to prepare such meals on their own without dependence on junk.

5. Role of Food Companies

Food companies also play a great role in awareness and transparency. Companies set out to embrace health and wellness can set a benchmark for other companies. Here's how the food companies can help:

Clean Labeling Practices: These companies should promise clear and accurate labeling practices, so that consumers are easily in the know about additives like maltodextrin and what they might cause.

Ingredient Transparency: Companies can ensure giving consumers actual information on sourcing practices, production methods, and even purposes for each ingredient, thereby helping build trust with consumers and furthering healthy lifestyles choices.

Product Reformulation: Manufacturers can reformulate their product to avoid or minimize the necessity of certain additives-a healthier alternative for consumers seeking to ensure they are not consuming maltodextrin.

6. Cultivating Healthy Eating Culture

Lastly, teaching and education aim towards initiating healthy eating cultures in our communities. By teaching people to include whole foods first, question processed products, and demand transparency, we ready an environment in which health is observed and sustained.

Community Support Groups: The societies created for experience-sharing on recipes and tips on how to steer clear of additives will bring pressure to change lifestyles and adopt a healthier view of living.

Local Resources: Provide a list of resources at the local level indicating where one could find farmer markets, health food markets, and nutritionists who embrace healthy dietary behaviors.

Conclusion

In this regard, education and awareness will play a very significant role in fighting the possible hazardous effects maltodextrin may pose on human health. Encouraging an educated culture concerning diet and nutrition and aiding initiatives to educate society can assist improve the capacity of people to care for their health and also to take part in campaigns against unrestrained practices by the food industry.

And so, let us appreciate what education, advocacy, and a stronger community do for us in better selection. Let's talk now about the future of food additives: trends, research, and innovations which perhaps will define our present food supply.

Chapter 14 : Future of Food Additives: Emerging Trends and Innovations

As understanding shifts concerning what a food additive really is, the food-producing and consuming landscape changes with it. For future food additives, this chapter takes it further towards trending, innovative research, and developments that alter the way people see and relate to their foods. Currently popular talk regarding health, sustainability, and transparency in the food world is also discussed.

1. Changing Consumer Preferences

Consumer attitudes towards food and health have changed dramatically over the last decades, with increasing concerns towards ingredients like maltodextrin. The core is overall increased awareness and thus for more and more reasons consumers demand healthier, more natural products which leads to a change in the food industry trends in terms of direction:

Clean Label Products Growth: Minimalistic ingredients and transparency in labeling are what most consumers seek these days. Then clean labelling is led by the transparent labelling process, which does away with all the confusion over additives that no consumer would ever need to know.

Select Whole Foods: A more health-conscious consumer is on us, and the wave of whole, unprocessed foods is here. This will force food manufacturing to rely not on additives and preservatives but on the integrity of the ingredients.

Growing Demand for Alternative Plant: Based Products: The arrival of a plant-based diet brings in new alternatives to the standard products. In reality, plant-based food carries fewer additives, and therefore it goes predominantly in the direction of whole foods.

2. Future Changes in Regulations

As more and more people enlighten the additive to foods, regulations on their usage are becoming more restricted. The following could be some of the possible future regulations that may drastically focus on the following:

Tight Labeling Requirements: The regulatory authorities may enforce tighter labeling requirements on foods such that consumers will have proper knowledge of additives present in the food and the effect it might have on health.

Health Effects Research: Continued studies on health effects of additives such as maltodextrin will likely cause regulatory bodies to question the "safe" classification and amount being added to foods.

Transparency Standards: Growing consumer preference for more disclosure on the origin of food and the process by which it is manufactured will likely create regulations that will challenge manufacturers to provide better information about what they put in their products.

3. Innovative Research and Technology

Emerging research and technologically developed innovations are some of the factors that have taken a toll on the future of food additives. Some of the trends or concepts that may possibly be developed in the near future include natural alternatives. This is basically because scientists have started discovering alternative, more natural ways of introducing synthetic additives. Some of these substitutions are plant-based thickening agents and preservatives obtained from fruit and vegetables instead of chemically synthesized in a lab. Sometimes what is sold as natural offers equivalent functional benefits without any accompanying health risk.

Microbiome Research: Once diet research better links diet to gut health, researchers may target particular additives for subsequent study of how they specifically affect the gut microbiome. Consumers will clearly know what additives to avoid in order to keep their guts healthy.

Food Biotechnology: New biotechnologies are likely to usher in foods with better nutritional profiles that contain lesser or no levels of additives. For example, engineered crops may eventually have innate resistance to spoilage and thus require less or no preservatives.

4. Sustainability and Environment

Because of the spate of growing environmental concerns, sustainability has entered the food additive fray. Some of the emerging trends around sustainability include:

Food Waste Reduction Innovative Preservation: Innovations under development that can conserve food longer without using synthetic preservatives through methods like high pressure processing and natural fermentation.

Sustainable Sourcing: Consumers further want to buy products sourced in some form of sustainability. This can include, for example, renewable-resource-derived or environmentally friendly production additives.

Vegetarian-based solutions. This is because the market has embraced more plant-based products that tackle not only health concerns but also the sustainability issue at large. In this respect, manufacturers might be nudged to reflect more on the use of alternatives based on these values.

5. Education and Advocacy

Educational messages will be of high priority in the future for food additives. Nothing should overstep the basis of decision-making regarding diet and industry practices out of their hands: consumers, communities, and organizations. Among the ways education and advocacy can help, for instance, are the following:

Informed Consumers : The consumers will have more healthy choices and more transparency from manufacturers when they learn more about food additives and health problems emerging with their use.

Research Activism: Further study of additive health issues informs legislation and practice within industry. This could be the foundation for advocacy groups that are interested in issues of nutrition and food safety.

Community Activism: Community education, healthy eating promotion, and sustainable food systems will promote a culture of awareness toward more responsible food choices.

6. Personal Responsibility and Informed Choices

As the consumer, the future of food additives rests in our hands. This can be ensured through our choices, making intelligent decisions about what goes into the body, and insisting on healthier options. How?

Learn about food brands and what they're doing to ensure you are choosing a product aligned with your health and sustainability values. Pushing open companies might just encourage the change you want to see.

Share Awareness: Share your findings with anyone you are personally connected with. This is a great way in which nutrition and health issues can nudge others to take action.

Start becoming thoughtful choices in choosing more natural food and less packaged food products with fewer additives. This is an intentional choice, and, in return, communicates to the manufacturer your preference.

One such reason for such a change would include: food additives, changed demands of the consumers, changes in the regulatory conditions, new innovations, a mounting concern for sustainability, and many others. Based on such knowledge of health effects of maltodextrin-based additives or other preservatives, this article will initiate the call for active action in propounding the need to change in the food industry and other eating habits to avoid the worst that unhealthy lifestyle habits can cause.

In the concluding chapter, we will gather and summarize all those important contents discussed in all the preceding chapters to wrap up the exploration on how maltodextrin has some hidden dangers with a call to action to the reader to take control of choices of diet and raise awareness for healthier food options.

Chapter 15 : Summary and Call to Action: Stepping into Health Control

As this final page of our investigative journey about hidden dangers of maltodextrin it is worth reviewing the significant findings we came across in the course of this book. We learned how deep in complexity food additives are and just how they could impact us through matters related to health, bringing forth a very relevant issue in making the right diet. In the last chapter, we will give a summary of some of the essential information and a call to action on readers to assume responsibility for their care and well-being.

1. Key takeaways on Maltodextrin

Maltodextrin is one of the most extensively used food additives that have been obtained from starch in a tremendous number of processed food products. With a variety of different roles including being a thickener, stabilizer, and sweetener, maltodextrin has raised health implications, and here are the key takeaways:

Digestive Problems: Malto-dextrin can interfere with gut health by disrupting the balance of the gut flora leading to digestive problems and so forth.

Effect on Blood Sugar: Due to its high glycemic index, maltodextrin can shoot blood sugar through the roof within no time, especially of much harm to a person having diabetes and insulin resistance.

Addictiveness and Cravings: Maltodextrin in processed snack food can cause addictive-type eating behaviors and craving for unhealthy foods.

2. Awareness is Important

Through the book, we have always highlighted the role of education and awareness in this issue. Education and awareness are the best ways to make informed food choices. Awareness of what goes into our foodstuff, for example, an additive called maltodextrin, is proactive health protection. The key messages about awareness are:

Ingredient Literacy: Understanding food labels and knowing harmful additives will give consumers healthy choice power.

Community Engagement: Educating communities on food additives and their health hazards can spur a community to stand up for healthy food intake.

3. Advocacy

Advocacy is very central in the Food System of the future. As consumers, we do demand from industry operations regarding such practices and labeling of food products. Key advocacy points include:

Demanding Transparency: We can be the change in the food industry by choosing to buy from companies that label transparently and only sell products that are made with integrity.

Participating in Policy Changes: Contacting local representatives and pushing hard for updated regulation on food additives will force them to implement meaningful alterations in food safety standards.

4. Informed Choices

As we near the end of our study on maltodextrin and its implications, we must all take personal responsibility for what we eat. Here are some action steps you can take:

Read Labels: Make it a habit to carefully read the food labels for your products. Become aware of products which minimize or have eliminated the use of additives such as maltodextrin.

Choose Whole Foods: Make whole, unprocessed foods the core of your diet. Focus on fresh fruits and vegetables, whole grains, lean proteins, and healthy fats.

Cook More: Cook meals from scratch using fresh ingredients as often as possible. This promotes healthier eating and a closer connection to the food.

5. Inspiring a Healthier Community

But individually, as persons, we can actually be the leaders in building a healthier community. Here are some tips on how to encourage other people's participation in the conversation about food additives and health:

Start Conversations: Discuss with friends and family the importance of ingredient awareness. Share stories and learnings from personal experiences to encourage others to make better choices.

Organize Community Events: Organize a workshop or cooking class or a health fair in your community as an opportunity for education on nutrition and food additives.

Advocate for Local Programs: Reach out to local groups or initiatives whose mandate is the facilitation of healthy eating promotion and nutrition education.

6. Your Action

Awareness, education, and action are the start of health improvement. As we close this book, we challenge you to do the following:

Learn More: Discover more and more about food additives and its health implications. Educate yourself on the latest research or trends regarding nutrition.

Be the Change: Take charge of your life and decide to eat smart. Eat more whole food and pay attention to what you eat.

Join Campaign: Join others who demonstrate openness about food labels and change better food in your community. Your voices can be very powerful, driving changes if you join forces.

Conclusion:

There is a hidden danger of maltodextrin and other such food additives, which we can never ignore. Knowing the possible health effects they might cause and how we can become proactive advocates for transparency and healthier choices, we'll pave our way towards a brighter future in nutrition.

As we incorporate these habits, let's not forget that every small decision in our diets builds toward an enduring enhancement in health and wellness. Let's commit ourselves to smart choices, resourcefulness, and advocacy for healthier foods in our environment, where everyone benefits from ease of access to nutritious, fresh foods that facilitate a healthier life.

Thanks for traveling with us. To a healthier tomorrow, one more informed choice at a time.

Chapter 16 : Conclusion and Future Directions

As we close this book, we are now geared to reflect on lessons learned while exploring maltodextrin in the context of food additives. We therefore sum up the major themes discussed, outline the long journey still ahead to healthy eating, and urge you to continue agitating for better food choices in your life and community.

1. Summary of Key Takeaways

From the pages above, it explained the subtlety of the word maltodextrin and then in detailing its impact on human health. Key points I note from above are as follows:

What is Maltodextrin: One must understand what this is, how it is produced, and how prevalent it is in the food products. We know this as an emulsifier and stabilizer/sweetener role in other foods.

Health Effects: In the previous section, some of the potential dangers of maltodextrin in the food group, including blood glucose influence, gut flora influence, and contribution to additive consumption patterns, were discussed.

Transparency Matters : Clear food additive labeling was the most important demand made by the labelers. Customers have a right to know what is in their food : power through knowing your food choices.

Community Involvement and Awareness: We also noted that community initiatives, awareness, and education on healthier eating and the interference of additives point to the best.

2. The Journey to Healthy Eating

While this book is a guide for the adventure in knowing the side risks hidden about maltodextrin, it still marks the beginning journey along the way towards a lifelong guide on healthy eating. Remember these key things on the way:

Small Changes Matter: New habits take time to establish. Create small, achievable changes in your diet. Each good decision adds up to the sum of your health.

Focus on Whole Foods: Eat whole, minimally processed food that optimally feeds your body. Focus on a variety of fruits, vegetables, whole grains, and lean proteins in your eating plan for an attempt at balance in your diet.

Keep Current: Nutrition science is constantly changing; understanding what is hot and what is coming will allow you to make good decisions. Read good resources, take workshops, and get in touch with professionals who are in the nutrition field.

3. Keeping the Conversation Alive

As you continue on your journey, it will be essential to keep the conversation about food additives and health. Here are ways to keep this dialogue:

Share Your Knowledge: Write down possible hazards of maltodextrin supplements for your friends and family to be aware of. Discussion of nutrition educates the public about what they are doing when they go out to get their food.

Utilize the social media on the internet: like blogs, Facebook, Twitter, etc. to share resources, articles, and personal experience concerning food additives and healthy eating. That will further expand your scope and connect you with others who hold similar views and have the same goal.

Get involved in locally operating initiatives: Join your neighborhood health groups, grow produce at the farmers' markets, or join a food co-op that supports healthy eating and sustainability. You can most definitely find using your community very helpful to an environment for making different choices.

4. Call to Action

Wherever consumers are, they can be advocates for a better way to approach food policies and practices. Here's how you can work to take your passion of healthy eating and make it advocacy:

Contact your representatives : Join your voices with those of local representatives on food labeling and harmful activities of harmful additives. Your voice may just dictate policy changes for your public health.

Help Organizations: Give time or money to any organization that's actively involved in nutrition education, food safety, or public health care. Collective action can surely bring a big change in food systems.

Connect to Community Health Initiatives: Connect with or create community health initiatives that are initiatives in nutrition education, food access, or healthy eating. Work together and magnify the effort.

5. Future

Not over yet is the debate of food additives, such as maltodextrin. These trends and developments would define our food supply as we step into the future:

Food Science Innovation: Now we can at least envision innovations on health and sustainability of food production that would more naturally replace the above harmful additives.

Higher level consumer awareness: More aware consumers of the quality of food and health will result in many companies being concerned over transparency, as well as reformulation of products for clean label requirements.

Global Movements: With healthier eating moving in every nook and corner of the world, the governments and the industries will be made not to succumb to those practices that line their pockets at the cost of public health.

Conclusion

Closing this, the silent killers maltodextrin and other food additives bring home the fact that vigilance over what we eat is paramount. The road to healthier eating calls for a commitment to learning, advocating, and building community amongst many things.

We thank you in advance for taking time out to learn with us from such important topics. Hopefully, our book will also have given you knowledge, information, and tools that can guide you toward healthy choices of food additives toward a healthier future.

Your choices matter. From today onward, become aware and knowledgeable of the choices that could well drive better changes-not just to your own lives but to others' lives as well. Let's rise to this future together so that all people, everywhere have safe and nutritious food and healthy diets.

Chapter 17 : Epilogue: Getting Closer to a Healthier Future

As we conclude this venture into the unknown threats of maltodextrin and generally about food additives, it's time to take this information shared further by pro-actively embracing a healthier journey. This journey to healthiness, concerning what we consume is incessant and fluid, representing one's personal choice as well as a community effort to move toward healthier lifestyles.

1. Empower Yourself and Others

In fact, knowing the effects of maltodextrin and other such additives gives you power to make sound decisions. You may even pass on this power to people around you. Here are some steps toward creating a healthy consciousness in people.

Be a Role Model: Encourage your family and friends to reconsider their eating habits by showing them the decisions you take towards a healthier lifestyle, including the setbacks and accomplishments.

Create Supportive Environments: This can happen at home, work, or even community groups. Host a potluck with whole foods or share recipes that are in line with clean eating principles.

Educate Future Generations: Teach children and young adults about the principles of nutrition and how to understand food labels. This will inform them of what they should be choosing as they grow up.

2. Creating Mindful Eating Behaviors

Mindful eating, therefore, can be incredibly beneficial for fostering healthier food relationships and leading to better health outcomes. How to be mindful when it comes to eating:

Eat More Slowly: Signals of Hunger And Satiety In Foods Low-calorie Retreat Meal use coverage Eating slows down your chewing so you can actually taste the food (imagine that) and, more importantly, feel full instead of shoveling far too much into your piehole obliterating any chance at hunger becoming satiety.

Listen to How Your Body Responds: Be mindful of how food makes you feel. Between the two, let your thinking guide you in what healthy foods to grab this week.

Give Thanks: Stop before a meal to reflect on what you have been given as nourishment. A habit of gratitude can provide a greater appreciation for nourishing options, while also reinforcing balanced perspectives on eating and health.

3. Community Involvement End

Act toward healthier eating by considering how you may help shape food environments through community engagement. Here's how you can get started:

Support Local Farmers: Purchase from a local farmers' market or sign up for a community-supported agriculture (CSA) program. This helps to support sustainable practices and provides you with the freshest, in-season produce.

Advocate for Food Justice: Engage with campaigns in your local community focused on food access and equity. Support campaigns to gain healthy food access for those who lack it.

Join Educational Workshops: Join or undertake workshops around you aimed at teaching the community on how to become nutritional experts and people who 'can read between the lines' when it comes to food labels.

4. Using Technology Better

In an information age, being that much better equipped to understand your food choices by virtue of the right technology by your side means you can do the following:

Use Technology Effectively for Proper Nutrition:

There are some of the best ways to use technology effectively for proper nutrition.

Track Food Intake Using Apps: To help track your nutritional intake and acquire plenty of insights regarding the content in your food as well as the quality of ingredients, consider using apps.

Keep Up with What's Happening Online: Pay attention to social media accounts of reputable nutrition experts and organizations and professional research institutions. That can keep you abreast of the latest information and tips on healthy choices.

Be an Active Online Community Member: You can be part of some online forums or social media groups that focus on healthy eating and advocacy; sharing experiences and resources fosters a real sense of community and support.

5. The Future of Nutrition

The future looks bright with a steady stream of innovation and momentum toward the trend of transparency and health in food and nutrition. Some of the trends and evolutions to look forward to in the near future include the following:

Food production technology: Studies in biotechnology and improved sustainable practices are likely to lead to healthier foods and fewer harmful additives.

A Steady Growth in Personalized Nutrition: Thus, it will be built along the lines of different individual health needs and genetic profiles. The growth in this area of personalized nutrition will be so designed to offer its consumers specific dietary recommendations that will yield better health outcomes.

Global Movements for Health Equity: Much awareness about food justice may force policymakers and businesses to act responsibly about disparities in access to healthy food.

Conclusion: A Personal Commitment to Health

As you close these pages, take a minute to reflect on your personal commitment to health and well-being. Every decision you make contributes to a much larger narrative regarding food, how we treat it, and how it affects our lives and the world around us.

Commit to being an informed consumer, advocate for transparency in food labeling, and encourage others to join the journey toward healthier eating. It's time to foster a culture doing the most for nutrition, sustainability, and health equity with all of us.

Thanks for shining your light so that it shines, keeping ahead on the radar screen of knowledge about the potential dangers posed by maltodextrin and other food additives. Wishing you a continued trail of inspiration and empowerment for you and those around you, for many years to come.

FAQs (Frequently Asked Question)

These are the most commonly asked questions about maltodextrin, food additives, and healthy eating. This could be a very useful reference for those interested in discovering more or just wanting to check facts they are unsure about.

1. What is Maltodextrin, and Where is it Found?

Maltodextrin is a carbohydrate that is produced from starch. It is found, therefore, as one of the modern, often highly processed foods such as fillers and thickeners or even as a preservative. Some product lines include:

Snack Foods: Chips, granola bars, and other snack foods contain maltodextrin to enhance texture and shelf life

Beverages: Some sports drinks and powdered drink mixes contain maltodextrin for sweetness purposes but also as a fast energy source.

Sauces and Dressings: Maltodextrin is a stabilizer which occurs in most of the sauces, salad dressings, and condiments.

Baked Goods: It is used in bread products along with other items in baked goods so that it may become soft and creamy due to retention of moisture.

2. Is Maltodextrin Safe to Eat?

Maltodextrin is generally recognized as a safe food additive by the FDA if consumed in moderate quantities. However, excessive consumption leads to various health problems such as

Blood Sugar Increases: Maltodextrin contains a very high glycemic index that may raise the blood sugar level in a very short time, particularly among diabetic patients.

Gut Health Problems: Some have stated that maltodextrin may lead to problems with gut bacteria, hence possibly resulting in stomach disorders

Addictive Food Intake: The sweet taste and palatability of food prepared with maltodextrin means its products cause overindulgence and more hunger for processed foods.

To verify if a food product contains maltodextrin, always check the ingredient list. Sometimes, maltodextrin is used and has another name such as:

1. **Maltodextrin**
2. **Dextrins**
3. **Starch hydrolysate**

Be wary of ingredient lists, especially for products labeled "low-calorie" or "sugar-free", because these products use maltodextrin in order to supplement the lost sugar.

4. What are some alternatives to maltodextrin?

If you want to avoid maltodextrin, consider these alternatives for thickening or sweetening:

Arrowroot Powder: a plant-based, natural thickener in sauces and soups

Agar-Agar: a plant-based gelling agent available as a replacement to maltodextrin in wide varieties of products.

Coconut Sugar: a lower glycemic index sweetener that can replace maltodextrin in specific products.

5.What can i do for honest food labeling and regulation?

Community-level action: advocate honest food labeling and regulation through policies by doing the following

Involve Your Members of the City Council: Contact your members of the City Council and request an opportunity to speak with them about your concern for the issue on food labelling and the use of dangerous additives.

Go to Public Hearings: Attend public forums or meetings regarding food safety and public health issues so you can express your views.

Engage in Advocacy Groups: Look for organizations with the same beliefs regarding food safety and nutrition. Advocacy groups, most of which have community mobilization resources, can be found.

6. What Role Does Education Play in Choosing the Right Diet?

Education aids individuals in making more discerning choices about diet. It can be interpreted through:

Ingredient Labels: The ability to read and understand food labels-this conditions the customers to read the additives in food, keeping them more informed with their choice.

Nutrition Science: A right footing in nutrition science will make an individual differentiate between adverts and scientific statements regarding food.

Culinary Skills: Gaining the skills for cooking will help a person prepare meals from whole ingredients, thus getting away from a diet of processed food.

Conclusion

It is through and within the food choices that one comes to realize knowledge is power. The knowledge gained regarding the implications of an ingredient such as maltodextrin could reshape the perspective that one has towards health and well-being. You have to encourage this proactive approach toward food literacy to empower your choices based on your health goals.

Moreover, your dedication to the understanding of food additives and promoting better practice goes beyond benefiting just you, but may also positively influence your community by discussing what you learned and supporting people around you, thus becoming part of a collective movement toward a healthier food environment.

Thanks for taking the time to engage with this content. May your journey to health and wellness inspire not just yourself but others around you, and together, we can build a future where healthy, safe, and wholesome food is the norm.

Glossary of Terms

Nutrition and food additives jargon will help you develop your ability in making informed decisions. Here's a glossary of terms regarding maltodextrin, food additives, and nutrition for you as you move on

1. Additive

These are substances added to food products in order to improve the taste, appearance or shelf life of the food product. Additives can either be of natural origin or synthetic

2. Carbohydrate

A macronutrient that gives the body energy. Carbohydrates can be distinguished into two types: simple-sugars and complex-starches and fibers.

3. Food Label

It is also known as a name given to packaged foods holding information about the product, what nutrition content is contained in that product, what ingredients make up that food, as well as serving sizes.

4. Glycemic Index (GI)

The period over which a carbohydrate-rich food elevates blood glucose level. The foods with high GI elevate the blood sugar concentration in the body very fast.

5. Hydrolysis

It is the chemical reaction that is used to break down complex molecules into simpler ones, sometimes starch is broken down into maltodextrin using it

6. Monosaccharide

This also is the simplest form of carbohydrates. It contains only one molecule of sugar. Examples of which are glucose and fructose.

7. Polysaccharide

It is a complex carbohydrate; containing many chains of monosaccharides. The examples of polysaccharides include starch and fiber.

8. Processed Food

It is that food, which has been changed from its original state; generally it contains several additives, preservatives, or artificial components in order to improve taste, texture, or shelf-life.

9. Natural Flavour

A term for flavouring developed from natural sources, like animals and plants, but the actual ingredients to be used are vague.

10. Whole Foods

Processed minimally so that no artificial additives and preservatives are added. This category includes fruits, vegetables, whole grains, nuts, and seeds.

Sample Weekly Meal Plan

In order to make it easy to transition into a balanced diet rich in whole foods and low on as few additives as maltodextrin, here's a sample menu for the day below.

Day 1

Breakfast: Sweet oat porridge topped with fresh berry toppings and honey drizzle

Lunch: Quinoa chickpeas salad, with chunks of cucumber, cherry tomatoes, and dressing mixed into it using lemon vinaigrette

Dinner: Grilled chicken breast with steamed broccoli and sweet baked potatoes

Snack: Almond butter with sliced apples

Day 2

Breakfast: Banana, spinach, and unsweetened almond milk smoothie

Lunch: Stir-fried vegetables with tofu and brown rice

Dinner: Baked salmon with asparagus, accompanied by quinoa

Snack time: Carrot sticks with hummus

Day 3

Breakfast: Greek yogurt, topped with walnuts and cinnamon

Lunch: Whole grain wrap with turkey, spinach, and avocado

Dinner: Stir-fried vegetable with shrimp, accompanied by brown rice

Snack time: Mixed nuts

Day 4

Breakfast: Scrambled eggs, spinach, and whole-grain toast

Lunch: Lentil soup salad.

Dinner: take one cup of cooked quinoa , beef and vegetable stir-fry only.

Snack: take one normal size of apple.

Day 5

Breakfast: For breakfast, soak some chia seeds and half a banana in a glass of almond milk and eat it after some time.

Lunch: Make a vegetable sandwich on whole grain bread in sufficient quantity and then eat it after grilled.

Dinner: Make a vegetable sandwich on whole grain bread in sufficient quantity and then eat it after grilled.

Snack: Take a bowl of yogurt and top it with granola and then eat it.

Day 6

Breakfast: First make a bowl of berry smoothie and then consume it after topping it with some granola.

Lunch: Salad containing spinach, nuts, cranberries with grilled chicken.

Dinner : Zucchini noodles with marinara and turkey meatballs.

Snack: Celery sticks with peanut butter.

Day 7

Breakfast: Soak oats overnight the day before, then mix almond milk, chia seeds, finely chopped peaches and eat it.

Lunch: For lunch, make a bowl of quinoa with black beans, some corn and avocado and eat it.

Dinner: Make a cabbage salad at night and eat it with grilled taco fish with avocado sauce.

Snack: Eat some air-popped popcorn as you can.

Conclusion

As you read through and experience what this book has in store for you, remember that every small step toward a healthier diet really packs that big wallop for overall wellness. It's not all about avoidance; it's embracing the lifestyle of whole, nutritious foods toward better health.

Feel free to use this glossary and this meal plan as a guide to help you make the right choice in nutrition and health; share it with others, and keep on discussing nutrition and health to achieve a more informed and healthy community.

Thank you so much for your dedication to the hidden dangers of maltodextrin and your stance on wellbeing above anything else. Only your journey has only just begun, and good things are ahead!

Thank you